21 Questions

About Cleanses

Answered

Daphne A. Caffe

DISCLAIMER

This information is solely for informational purposes. IT IS NOT INTENDED TO PROVIDE MEDICAL ADVICE. Neither the editors, the author, nor publisher take responsibility for any possible consequences from any treatment, procedure, exercise, dietary modification, action or application of medication which results from reading or following the information contained in this book. The publication of this information does not constitute the practice of medicine, and this information does not replace the advice of your physician or other health care provider. Before undertaking any course of treatment, the reader must seek the advice of their physician or other health care provider.

Connect to the Network

Web ~ Delightfullypleasure.me

Facebook.com/delightfulp

Twitter ~ DlightflPleasrs

Soundcloud.com/delightfulpleasures

Instagram: Delightfullypleasure.me

Table of Contents

Introduction

It seems like cleanses are all of the rage these days. Our friends and our family might be speaking about a cleanse they just did or are planning on doing. There is regular media coverage on new cleanses. Master Cleanse! Raw food Cleanse! Green Smoothie Cleanse! We are being peddled cleanses on T.V. and in our shopping malls. Lose weight! Feel great! Get an energy boost! Remove dangerous toxins! Cure cancer! The hype raises many questions. What is a cleanse? How do you cleanse? What are the benefits of cleansing? What are some types of cleanses? In this book I will answer all of these questions and many more. By the end of the book you will have a solid foundation on cleansing.

I will begin by answering the question, "What is with the hype surrounding cleanses?" The hype is that with all of the toxins our bodies come into contact with every single day, we are becoming a nation of very unhealthy people. Toxins can be absorbed into our bodies in many ways, including the foods we eat, the water we drink, and the air we breathe. Toxins are poisons to our systems that can damage tissues and cause many health-related symptoms. Chemicals can be toxic and seep into our bodies through the air, our food, or water. Pesticides, second hand cigarette smoke, and pollution can all be toxic to the human body.

Body cleanses are about resting, cleaning, and nourishing the body. Detoxification begins by eliminating the poisons from the body, then nourishing it with healthier foods. A body cleanse can help prevent disease and help the body stay healthy. Eating the right foods after a total cleansing of the body will ensure the results will last.

Toxins in the body could be responsible for the tired feeling so many people report having every day of their lives. The poisons could also be causing headaches, intestinal problems, anxiety, nerve disorders, sleeplessness, depression, and mood disorders. Toxins may even be responsible for some birth defects.

On the other hand, all of these health problems have been around for as long as people have. It is hard to say whether the problem is greater now than ever or just reported more often as people have an easier time getting health care for minor annoyances. Some of the reports on the dangers of the toxins we are exposed to come from companies who are trying to sell their cleanses so it can be very difficult to know who or what to believe. The news is enough to scare people into trying anything to get rid of the poisons in their bodies.

Hype established, I am going to answer 21 questions that you might have about cleanses. In this book you will find foundational information on cleansing with some interesting tidbits that may lead you to further research.

Q1 ~ What is a Body Cleanse?

The purpose behind performing a cleanse is to remove harmful toxins from the body. Many different types of cleanses exist, including ones to cleanse the physical body, the mind, and the spirit. There are several types of body cleanses that can be done at home, either with purchased cleanse regimens or from products that can be made at home.

Certain types of cleanses involve drinking only fruit juices or water for several days to allow the digestive system to clear itself of everything. With other cleanses, people are instructed to use laxatives to clean out their systems and still others involve eating only certain foods, such as fruits and vegetables, for several days. With these special diets some people report withdrawal symptoms such as headaches, nausea, and weakness. Hunger is also an important consideration before choosing a diet based cleanse. It is often believed that the only way to perform a body cleanse is by what is eaten or drank, but there are other types of cleanses. Some can be done by massage, others by meditation, and still others by using gels or creams to draw toxins from the body.

I will discuss all of these topics in further detail later in the book.

Many people perform body cleanses when they begin to feel sluggish or rundown. Others plan a body cleanse at the same time every month or every few months to prevent toxins from building up in their body. People who believe in a holistic way of life firmly believe that body cleanses are necessary for a healthy body.

Q2 ~ What is the History of Cleanses?

The process of purifying the body goes back for centuries. Historians have found written documents from ancient China that date back to 2700 B.C. that show how to perform a body cleanse. Historians have also found that as long ago as 400 B.C, people cleansed their bodies by eliminating certain foods and eating a plant-based diet. Cleansing often began as part of a religious ritual. Native Americans often performed purification, by fasting or by ingesting herbs, as part of their religious practice. They believed that they could more easily commune with the natural world and the Gods that guided their lives when they had purified their bodies.

Herbs and other plants have been used for centuries to clean out different organs of the body, such as the colon, liver and kidneys. Because these organs are so vital to removing toxins from our bodies, it was believed that keeping them clean and healthy was the most important thing a person could do to stay healthy.

People of ancient Greece and Egypt believed in auto-detoxification. This is a way of eating that encourages the body to cleanse itself. Many of the beliefs that were held in those long ago days are

still believed today, such as eating a plant based
diet and drinking plenty of water.

Q3 ~ Why Should I Cleanse?

We no longer live in a natural world. Chemicals, pollution, and poisons have pervaded our environment. These toxins are all around and seep into the body in many different ways. Everything that is eaten can contain toxins and so can the water that is consumed. Even the air has poisons in it that can harm the body. A body cleanse can be used to detox the body and remove the toxins that the body cannot get rid of itself.

When people hear the word toxin they might think of poison and become scared. These poisons are not likely to kill a person themselves, but they can cause real harm to the body as they aggregate. Too many toxins in the body can cause a person to feel many different ways. Skin problems, such as acne, or hair that is too brittle can be a result of too many toxins. A change in sleeping patterns or having little or no appetite can also be the result of high toxicity in the body. Nagging headaches, allergies, or sinus problems could also be caused by the toxins that have gathered in the body.

Body cleanses are used to remove the excess toxins from the body to bring the body back to a healthy state. A healthier body can fight off diseases and infections much easier. People who feel better are more likely to eat right and exercise which in turn brings about more positive results. Bodies with fewer toxins are more likely to fight off cancer, heart disease, and other dangerous health concerns.

One reason so many people use body cleanses is that it is easy and nearly anyone can do it. Of course, it is important to discuss body cleanses with a physician before doing one to be safe. Some doctors firmly believe in the detoxification of the body while others are not so sure. Most agree that it cannot hurt, but before doing a detoxification, talk to a physician. If you are planning on doing a cleanse that calls for the ingesting of herbs and you take any types of medication you should be especially careful and discuss your plans with a physician. Herbs and medications can have terrible reactions to each other that could be dangerous.

Body cleanses tend to become more popular after the Christmas holiday season when people are feeling especially stuffed and tired. With so many celebrations and parties, it is easy to over-indulge on food and alcohol. People are also a lot more rushed during that time of year and tend to eat more fast food and get less sleep. Exercising also takes a back seat to everything else that needs to be done. By the beginning of the New Year the excess and over-indulgence has many people feeling sluggish and depressed. A body cleanse can help alleviate those feelings and restore the body. Weight gain can be controlled, or even reduced, after doing a body cleanse and people often report feeling brighter and happier. These feelings encourage a healthier lifestyle and help fight the post-holiday blues.

Another popular time for people to reach for body cleanses is late spring when they start thinking about bathing suit weather and vacations. Body cleanses can help tighten the skin on the body and help get rid of the weight that was gained over the winter. By spring, many people are feeling "winter blahs" and doing something as simple as a body cleanse to get ready for spring and summer can help brighten their moods.

Q4 ~ Are there Dangers to Body Cleansing?

Despite the popularity of cleanses, some of them can be harmful to the body. Cleanses that call for repeated fasting or only drinking liquids can be especially hard on the human body. If the chosen cleanse involves herbs, be aware of reactions between the herbs and any medications that may be taken. It is also possible to flush out the good bacteria in the human body with a cleanse.

With any type of cleanse that involves repeated or long-term fasting; many experts are concerned about possible vitamin deficiencies that can occur when the body is not given the fuel it needs to maintain good health. The human body needs a specific balance of vitamins, minerals, and proteins to work as it should. When these items are taken away, the deficiency can cause the body to start breaking down muscles to get the nutrients it needs. Blood-sugar problems can also become a problem when fasting occurs often or over a long period of time. In the process of trying to become healthier, people who frequently fast can actually be inviting more health problems. When the body does not have the nutrients it needs, it also becomes harder to fight off infections and illnesses. A balance of nutrients needs to be maintained for the best overall health and even a small fluctuation can be a problem.

Anyone who takes medications should talk to their doctor before attempting any cleanse that involves herbs. Medications and herbs can react against each other and may be especially dangerous. Many body cleanses are available that do not involve using herbs. If medications are taken an herb-free option might be the safer option.

Some doctors raise the concern that fasting or juice only body cleanses can actually harm the body by removing vital good bacteria from the intestines. Many doctors feel that the kidneys, liver, and intestines do an excellent job of removing toxins from the body and fasting to remove toxins is an unnecessary risk. The human body has many types of good bacteria and either fasting or an all liquid body cleanse runs the risk of flushing this vital bacteria from the body. Losing this bacteria can cause the body's natural flushing system – the kidneys, liver, and intestines – to work improperly. If they are not working properly the body will be unable to remove toxins efficiently and this can cause more health problems than the person had before the cleanse.

People can encourage the growth of bacteria in the body by taking probiotics and eating fermented foods such as pickled vegetables or soy products. Eating yogurts is also an excellent way to grow helpful bacteria in the digestive system. With the right amount of bacteria in the body, the digestive system will be able to flush toxins easier.

Another possible danger is that severe calorie restrictions over a long period of time can cause headaches, irritability, and body pains. These are often exactly what people are trying to get rid of by performing a cleanse. Some fasting cleanses require the use of laxatives which can cause even more problems like dehydration.

Pregnant women, older adults, and anyone with kidney or heart disease should be extremely careful if they want to try to attempt a body cleanse. The danger may be too great for any benefit that might occur. People with digestive disorders should also avoid fasting because of the danger of a flare up of the disease.

The body is made up mostly of water and dehydration can be devastating. The body needs plenty of fluids so that it can function as it should. Organs need a lot of water to remove toxins and waste products from the food that is ingested each day. Before attempting any type of cleanse preparations need to be made to ensure that proper hydration is maintained throughout the entire cleanse. Juices and green teas are healthy fluids, but water is the best option for keeping fluid levels adequate during the cleanse. Soda drinks and coffee actually dehydrate the body so these are not good choices to keep the body hydrated.

Q5 ~ What are Some Different Types of Body Cleanses?

When most people think of a body cleanse, a water-only or juice-only cleanse is often what they think of. While these are certainly very popular choices, there are many other types of body cleanses. A vegetable or fruit only diet is a choice, as is fasting for several days or several times a month. There are pills available that are supposed to help flush toxins from the body and some people use laxatives to completely flush their intestines.

For people who are concerned about changing their diet so drastically, there are other options for a body cleanse. Gels or creams can be purchased to be used topically and draw toxins from the body through the skin. Meditation is an option as is massage therapy. Many people feel that anything that will help reduce the stress the body feels will flush toxins from the body. Some people argue that even exercise can have a cleansing effect among its other health benefits. Before any exercise program is started, be sure to consult a doctor.

Yoga and pilates are also considered to be useful body cleanses. Ancient civilizations believed a true purification of the body could not occur until the mind, body, and spirit were one. Yoga and pilates both offer exercises that are meant to strengthen and tone the body while the slow, gradual position changes encourage the mind and spirit to relax and become quiet. Some experts feel that the true toxin in the body is the stress that so many people live with each day. To truly cleanse the body, stress relieving techniques can be considered a great way to start.

Q6 ~ What is a Juice Cleanse?

For many people an easy body cleanse is one that can be performed over a weekend and includes drinking a lot of juice and little else. The idea is that the diet of only juice will clean out the body and remove any potentially dangerous toxins that may be lingering in the body. Even some medications do not flush from the body and a cleanse can help remove them.

A juice cleanse can be a way to clear out the toxins in the body or a way to introduce a new, healthier way of providing nutrients to the body. A juice cleanse can take a little preparation. About three days before the cleanse, make sure to drink eight glasses of water each day and slowly eliminate bad foods from your diet, such as soda, fast food, and junk foods. This will help adjust the body to the smaller amount of food that is consumed during a juice cleanse.

ACTION PLAN: For a juice cleanse, start with an eight ounce glass of water with half of a lemon squeezed into it and then drink six eight ounce servings of juice throughout the day. If hunger becomes a problem you can have more servings. If the hunger persists eat a small portion of raw vegetables, such as carrots or avocados. Be aware of any odd symptoms the body may be having and limit exercise to walking or stretching because the energy levels in the body will be much different during a juice body cleanse. Plan relaxing activities, such as reading or mediation, during the body cleanse so the mind and spirit can clear themselves as well. Be aware that the ears may become more sensitive to sounds during the juice cleanse and plan activities accordingly.

For several days following a juice cleanse, avoid anything too strenuous to allow the energy levels to rise in the body. Gradually add foods back into the diet, but choose ones that are easy to digest. Many companies sell prepared juice cleanses, but they can be expensive. If the person choosing the juice cleanse has little time this may be the way to go. A little thought can make preparing juice at home just as easy and much healthier. A blender and juicer would be great to have at home to prepare juices as they are needed. Smoothies are always a great way to continue the healthy diet after the juice cleanse has been completed. There are countless recipes on the web for different healthy juices and smoothies.

Q7 ~ What are Some Ideas for Smoothies and Detox Drinks?

It is easy to find information on possible recipes for juice detoxifications. Often, total body cleanses require a jump start drink to the day. Different green teas or flavored waters are often used to get the body cleanse started each day. Juices and smoothies created from various fruits such as pineapple, mango, pomegranate and lemons are popular drinks to create each morning. They are also easy to pack for a busy morning. Many juices can be made the night before but for the best nutrients, juices and smoothies should be consumed soon after they are made.

One popular juice is a vegetable juice with many colors of vegetables in it. The more colorful the ingredients are before they are mixed, the healthier the juice will be. For example, a juice created from tomatoes, carrots, lemons, and celery would be red, orange, yellow, and green. A juice created from a wide variety of colorful foods makes an awesome body cleanse juice that is very healthy too.

Turmeric, ginger, lemon juice, and cayenne pepper is another popular juice for people performing body cleanses. The turmeric is great for helping the liver detoxify and the ginger, lemon, and cayenne pepper all help the body remove dangerous toxins. Smoothies are a favorite way to start the day as they are more filling than juices and help hold off hunger pains. One delicious way to start the day and cleanse the body at the same time is create smoothies with any type of berries. Raspberries, blueberries, strawberries, and cherries are all delicious in smoothies. Blend any choice of berries with almond milk, flaxseed and some ginger for a terrific smoothie to start a body cleanse and keep the stomach full until mid-morning snack time.

Q8 ~ What is an example of a Diet Cleanse?

One of the most popular types of cleanses is a change in diet. When a diet cleanse is attempted the goal is to reduce the food the digestive system has to deal with while still making sure the body has sufficient fuel to function as it is supposed to. The purpose is to allow the body to perform its natural functions optimally, which includes cleansing the body of toxins, rather than having to deal with digesting an overload of food. This is a much less intense option than fasting because the body is still getting fuel, but the focus is still on letting the body do the work.

When a person is performing a body cleanse through their diet, the most common procedure is to only consume fruits, vegetables, juice from these, and plain water. It is much more natural for the body to digest fruits and vegetables than it is too digest highly processed and preserved foods. It is also easier for the body to digest fruits and vegetables than meats and dairy products. For these reasons fruits and vegetables form the basis of a dietary cleanse. As mentioned above, becoming dehydrated is a dangerous possible side-effect of cleanses. Anyone who attempts a dietary cleanse should drink plenty of water and juices made from fruits or vegetables. Fruits and vegetables are full of water and are and important part of most cleanses.

To get ready for a drastic dietary cleanse it can be wise to take some time to prepare the body. If a person typically consumes coffee, salt, sugar, animal products, or alcohol, they should take time to reduce how much of each they consume. While the body cleanse will work if they do not reduce their consumption, the withdrawal symptoms they may experience may cause them to stop the cleanse. Withdrawal symptoms can include headaches, nausea, and lightheadedness. Another preparation could be to remove the temptation of non-cleanse foods from the house and to stock up on fruits and vegetables.

Organic fruits and vegetables are an excellent option but it is not necessary to purchase only organic. If possible, choose foods that are in season to get the freshest choices. You can use almost any fruit or vegetable you enjoy during the dietary cleanse. Some of the best options include: citrus fruits, berries, grapes, coconut, plums, peaches, apples, bananas, pears, melon, squash, yams, potatoes, cabbage, lettuce, cucumbers, tomatoes, celery, carrots, peppers, broccoli and cauliflower. The body can easily digest each of these and it will not disrupt the body cleansing process. I will further discuss the benefits of certain foods in a future section. Hundreds of recipes are available to help people prepare new and different juice blends to keep their dietary cleanse from being too boring and causing them to reach for a bag of chips or a bottle of soda.

ACTION PLAN: The fruit and vegetable body cleanse is an easy one for most people. To begin, eat as many fruits and vegetables for breakfast as needed to feel full. An avocado can help the stomach stay full until lunch. A large salad can be prepared for lunch that includes as many vegetables as desired. If needed, eat a steamed potato after the salad to stay full until supper. Remember to drink water throughout the day. For supper plan to eat any combination of fruits and vegetables as desired but make sure to consume as many vegetables as fruits. Snacks throughout the day can be raw fruits and vegetables or smoothies created from them. If chewing foods is a problem, a blender can be used to mash the foods into softer servings. Whether the foods are chewed or mashed will not matter in the cleanse process.

This type of diet is perfect for a weekend cleanse or as a way to completely change the way a person eats. Withdrawal symptoms such as headaches and tiredness may be felt, and can be very strong, during the first few days. Often, after a few days, most people start to feel better. If other foods are going to be reintroduced into the diet, it should be done slowly, such as a serving of fish or eggs in the evening. Depending on how your body reacts, you can slowly increase servings and serving sizes if desired.

Often people report feeling so much better when they change their diet for a cleanse they change their eating habits permanently. An all plant-based diet can be very healthy but protein intake may be a concern. If a plant-based diet is going to be permanent, be sure to find a way to add protein to the diet in order to stay healthy. If you want to try to be a strict vegetarian lentils, beans, nuts, soy, seeds, and hemp are all options to getting the protein that the body needs. Otherwise, lean chicken, fish, and eggs are all easy ways to add protein to a diet.

Q9 ~ Can a Raw Food Cleanse Really Clear the Body of Toxins?

The hardest things for the body to digest and flush out are heavy fats and starches. The fast foods that many people seem to survive on are full of everything the body has a hard time cleaning out of the digestive system. It may seem to be too dramatic to try a raw food cleanse, but giving the body a rest from the onslaught of unhealthy foods can help it cleanse itself of the poisons that are making people sick each day.

A raw food diet can be extremely hard to follow, especially to those who feel they will not get full or who do not have time to prepare for it. One of the most important reasons to try a raw food body cleanse is the ease of preparation and the almost non-existent side effects. Beyond feeling hungry, with possible headaches due to that, the raw food diet is safe for most people. There are no pills to swallow and no herbs that may react with any medications that are being taken.

ACTION PLAN: To prepare for a raw foods body cleanse, a person needs to write a list of all fruits and vegetables that are liked and can be consumed raw. Nuts and seeds are also acceptable, if they are not salted or roasted. Some people even consume honey that is raw and locally produced, as to be sure it has not been processed. Water is a very important part of the diet to help the body feel full. The water can be flavored with ginger, lime, cucumber or mint to add variety to the diet. Generally the only maxim for a raw food diet is to eat as many raw fruits and vegetables as you need to feel satisfied. Fruits and vegetables are so low in calories and high in nutrition there is no need to calorie count or be overly restrictive of your intake.

To give the raw food cleanse time to flush the toxins from the body, plan to follow the diet for at least 5 days. Remember that any fruit or vegetable can be eaten on this diet and plan to mix and match each to be creative about tastes and what tastes good together. Salads are easy ways to use raw vegetables and can be prepared ahead of time. It would be rare that you can find raw salad dressing to add, but a little lemon or raw olive oil can be sprinkled over it. Broccoli and carrots are easy to pack and make excellent choices for a mid-afternoon snack.

Pecans and other nuts can add a little variety to the raw food cleanse and can also help the body feel full longer. Fruit salads make great snacks for when the body is craving something sweet. Plan to drink plenty of water and remember that an all raw food diet with a lot of water can make trips to the bathroom a frequent need.

A raw food body cleanse allows the body time to flush out dangerous toxins from the digestive system. Because these foods are so much easier to digest than meats, heavy starches and fatty foods, it gives the body a rest and time to work on getting rid of those poisons. Not only are raw vegetables and fruits easy on the body, they are full of the vitamins and minerals that so many people are desperately missing in their every day diets.

Following a raw foods body cleanse can easily become a habit. Even if a person adds small amounts of meat or proteins to the diet, it is a good possibility that weight loss will occur and illnesses will become fewer. Fruits and vegetables are low in calories and many are mostly water. This allows a person to feel full and still lose weight in a healthy, controlled way.

Body sugar and cholesterol levels are more easily controlled by this type of diet as well.

People with digestive problems or other health issues should consider following a raw foods diet to keep their body clean. If there you have health problems, talk to a physician before changing the diet so dramatically. People who choose to follow a raw food diet will not be as likely to need a total body cleanse in the future.

Q10 ~ What is the Master Cleanse?

The Master Cleanse has thousands of people who firmly believe that it helps them lose weight and get rid of the toxins in the body. However, there is scant scientific proof that the Master Cleanse does either. It is a juice fast that has been slightly modified. To begin, people on the Master Cleanse are not allowed to eat any food during the cleanse. Then instead of juices, they drink a specially prepared lemonade. The lemonade is made with two tablespoons of juice from an organic lemon (usually half a lemon will work for this), two tablespoons of maple syrup that is organic and grade B (cannot use the syrup most people use on pancakes), and one tenth of a teaspoon of cayenne pepper. Add each of these ingredients to ten ounces of filtered water and stir. Those are the ingredients for a typical serving. On average people will drink 4-8 pints of this lemonade concoction throughout each day they are on the cleanse. It is recommended that people go on the cleanse for roughly 10 days for the best results. Though, it is common do this cleanse for a weekend.

People who believe in the Master Cleanse say it removes toxins and excess fat from the body.

It can aid with temporary weight loss. What often happens is that when the person on the cleanse goes back to eating as they used to, the weight will come back. A cleanse itself is not the end of the story. To remain healthy one must maintain a healthy diet and exercise regularly.

While the Master Cleanse may be safe for a very short period of time, it may still cause headaches, dizziness, nausea, dehydration and fatigue. Anyone who decides to do a Master Cleanse of the body should plan ahead to be sure they can take it easy during the cleanse. Long term use of the Master Cleanse can have dangerous side effects, such as a loss of muscle mass. The Master Cleanse is not designed as a long term weight loss solution and special care should be taken when deciding to try this cleanse.

Many nutritionists call the Master Cleanse a crash diet and firmly believe it is an unhealthy way to detoxify the body or to lose weight. The lemonade mix is devoid of all the types of needed protein, minerals, and vitamins that the body requires to function properly. The long term effects cannot be measured easily and many experts would advise against doing the Master Cleanse for an extended period.

Q11 ~ How Do Specific Body Parts Cleanse The Body And Can They Be Cleansed?

The human body has an amazing system to eliminate waste. Sometimes there is too much waste or toxins that have accumulated and they are not easily removed from the body. Some people believe that each organ of the body needs their own cleanse in order for the body to be truly healthy. Some doctors do not believe this is necessary or even possible because the body works as an integrated whole, but for people who fully believe in the need for body cleanses, cleansing each organ is vitally important. There do appear to be some things you can do to help parts of your body function more efficiently. No matter what you believe, it is interesting to know the cleansing functions of different parts of the body.

Liver

The liver is the largest gland in the body and does a multitude of things. It works to take toxins from the blood, produces red blood cells, produces bile to digest fats, and stores iron and various vitamins. The liver regulates blood composition and works to remove any toxins that are in the blood before the blood leaves the liver for other parts of the body. Because the liver has so many functions, it is very important to keep it healthy. There are many foods that help cleanse the liver to keep it functioning properly. Among these super foods are beets, tomatoes, citrus fruits, cabbage, carrots, spinach, walnuts, apples, avocados, broccoli, and asparagus. Spices can be used to help clean out the liver, too, such as turmeric and garlic. Drinking green teas and using olive oil can also help the liver cleanse itself.

Kidneys

The kidneys are other organs that help remove waste from the body. Most of this is done by urination so drinking plenty of fluids helps the kidneys function as they are supposed to. Every day, they remove up to two quarts of water from foods that are consumed. Most experts agree that kidneys do not need any extra cleansing, as long as a person takes in enough water from liquids and foods that are eaten, such as fruits and vegetables. However, for those people who believe each organ needs to be cleansed, there are ways to cleanse the kidneys. Several companies market pills or drinks that claim to cleanse the kidneys. The safety of some of these products has been questioned.

For anyone who wants to prepare their own kidney cleanse, using herbs is a very popular way to start. Many herbs have qualities that aide in removing toxins from the kidneys, such as dandelion, nettles, goldenrod, ginger, parsley and marshmallow root. These herbs can be sprinkled over food or made into teas.

Colon

Doctors do not recommend cleansing the colon unless it is in preparation for a medical procedure. In that case, the physician will give specific instructions on how to prepare for the cleanse. There are many ways to keep the colon healthy that are not dangerous to the body. The easiest one is to eat properly and let the body take care of itself. To maintain a healthy colon, eat plenty of apples, avocados, spinach, cabbage, celery, flax and chia seeds. Each of these super foods contains nutrients that will help keep the colon clean.

If a person truly feels the need to cleanse the colon, there are many products available for sale. Be sure to carefully read the warning labels on any product that is chosen and follow the directions exactly as written. The colon can cleanse itself and does not really need a super cleansing unless recommended by a physician.

Skin

The largest organ of the human body is the skin. It absorbs toxins from the air every day and is often a place where toxins that are not removed from the body through the digestive system end up. Extra weight around the middle of the body can be caused by toxins lying near the skins surface. Eating healthy will help the skin, but there are also different products designed to remove those toxins through the skin.

Many body creams and gels are available to help pull out the toxins. There are several types and each person will need to choose the one that is best for them. One type is a cream that is rubbed onto the body at night and removed the next morning. Others involve adding a prepared liquid to a hot bath and soaking for thirty minutes. Another one is a gel that is rubbed onto the body and then plastic wrap is used to keep the gel tightly against the skin for as long as the person wants. Many people have reported exciting numbers of inches lost around their body after using products such as these. However, many of these are extremely expensive and experts believe the inches lost are actually water loss and not permanent. Again, these products need to be carefully researched and the directions followed carefully. Recipes are also available that can be prepared at home for use in the bath. These may be cheaper and healthier than purchased products.

Stomach

Enzymes that are produced in the stomach break down all food that is digested and helps to remove any potentially dangerous toxins that may have been ingested. Often, in the late spring, people see that their stomach is not as flat as they would like and reach for a stomach cleanse to achieve the desired sexy belly. However, a stomach cleanse will probably not be enough to ensure the stomach becomes and stays flat. Only proper nutrition and plenty of exercise will achieve the desired results. To jump start a new diet, a stomach cleanse can be used, but remember that stomach cleansings will cause the need for a bathroom to be close by at all times. Be sure to plan ahead before beginning any stomach cleanse. A one to three day fast is often the first thing recommended for a stomach cleansing, followed by using the cleansing product and increasing exercise. Remember that energy levels in the body will be lower due to the fast, so do not overdo the strenuous workouts.

Lungs

Many people do not think about their lungs when they consider a body cleanse. However, the lungs are constantly assaulted by mold, pollution, dust, and many other harmful things in the air every day. People who have quit smoking often want to cleanse their lungs to help them heal faster from the harmful aspect of smoking. Herbs are often used to cleanse the lungs because they can be an expectorant to help cough up the congestion in the lungs. Herbs can also soothe airways when they become irritated and can help relax muscles to calm bouts of coughing. Herbs can even fight organisms that can cause problems in the respiratory system.

Any of the following herbs can be used to help clear the lungs from harmful toxins. Osha root has been used for hundreds of years to aid the respiratory system. It contains camphor and increases the circulation to the lungs which allows deeper breaths. Many people already use various products with eucalyptus to help with respiratory problems. This herb is an expectorant, fights congestion and helps sooth irritated airways. It even boosts the immune system to help fight colds or flu. Peppermint is another very popular herb that people reach for when they have respiratory problems. Peppermint is so strong that even candy that is flavored with peppermint can open airways and fight congestions.

Q12 ~ What Specific Foods can Help Cleanse the Body?

Many foods can help the body cleanse itself. With fatty foods so readily available, it can be tough to eat properly each day. The foods below can help optimize the functions of different parts of the body. If they function properly they are able to clean themselves and the need for a total body cleanse becomes less likely. In fact, eating healthy can definitely prevent the need for a drastic total body cleanse.

- **Apples** contain phlorizin which stimulates bile production and helps the liver detoxify itself. Apples are also full of fiber and that helps pulls additives from foods and metals from the body. It is advisable to eat only organic apples because other types are in the top twelve foods that contain the most pesticides.

- **Artichokes** help with the production of bile in the liver. This allows the liver to cleanse itself of the toxins that can build up in it.

- **Avocados** are quickly becoming a super food because they contain antioxidants and help lower the cholesterol in the body while dilating the blood vessels. They also have a nutrient that can block many different types of carcinogens. Besides helping cleanse the liver, the list of benefits from eating avocados includes lower body weight and higher good cholesterol levels.

- **Beets** help the body cleanse itself by making sure the toxins that are removed actually leave the body. They purify the blood and help clean the liver. Beets also help fight infections.

- **Blueberries** contain detoxifying super-nutrients called proanthocyanidins. These berries are also full of antibiotics to prevent bacteria or toxins from gathering in the urinary tract.

- **Brazil Nuts** are vitally important in getting mercury removed from the body.

- **Basil** contains many antioxidants to protect the liver. It helps rid the body of toxins that build up because it is a diuretic that aides in flushing out the kidneys.

- **Broccoli** and broccoli sprouts aid the enzymes in the liver to convert poisons into something that can be easily eliminated from the body.

- **Cabbage** is another food that helps the liver cleanse itself. It also helps the body go to the bathroom regularly which in turn helps the entire body rid itself of toxins.

- **Cilantro** is one of the few foods that help remove metals from tissues so it can attach to other toxins and be flushed from the body.

- **Cranberries** have been proven to remove many different types of toxins from the body.

- **Dandelions** are very helpful to cleanse the liver and pancreas of poisons in the bloodstream. They are also helpful in cleansing the digestive tract in the body.

- **Flaxseeds** are vitally important when detoxing the body. The fiber in the flaxseed binds to toxins and helps to flush them from the intestinal tract of the body. Men need to be cautious when consuming flaxseed as it can mirror the effects of estrogen on the body.

- **Garlic** is included in almost all body cleanses because it helps the liver remove built up toxins from it. There is a lot of sulfur in garlic and sulfur is an excellent detoxifying food.

- **Ginger** can be added to hot water for a tasty tea or the root can be chewed on. It is important in cleansing the liver of alcohol or fatty foods.
- **Grapefruit** boosts the function of the liver and is full of nutrients that help other glands work to their fullest potential.
- **Green Tea** is included in almost all total body cleanses because it is full of antioxidants and helps with removing poisons from the body.
- **Hemp** is full of antioxidants and is vitally important in removing heavy metals from the body. It also helps keep the digestive tract clean.
- **Kale** boosts the body's ability to cleanse itself every day and prevents a buildup of toxins in the body's organs.
- **Lemongrass** has been used for centuries to cleanse the kidneys, bladder, liver, and the whole digestive tract. It is most often made into a tea for a total body cleansing.

- **Lemons** are often part of total body cleanses because the help change toxins into a water soluble form that can easily be removed from the body. Lemons are especially helpful in cleansing the liver.

- **Olive Oil** is another ingredient often used in body cleanse recipes. It helps the liver cleanse itself of toxins and to expunge any gallstones.

- **Onions** can be used to gather the mercury, lead, arsenic, and cadmium that can be in foods that are consumed daily. This vegetable also boosts the liver's ability to remove built up toxins.

- **Parsley** is full of all types of nutrients that protect the bladder and kidneys and enables them to cleanse themselves every day.

- **Pineapples** have an enzyme that cleans the colon when it is consumed. It also helps improve digestion and that aids in the body's ability to remove the toxins each day.

- **Seaweed** is rarely thought of as a food, but it has an amazing ability to bind to radioactive toxins that get into the body through food that has been grown where the soil has been contaminated. It can also help remove heavy metals that are hard to remove from the body and are especially dangerous to a healthy body.

- **Watercress** is an amazing food to help the liver perform its own cleansing.
- **Wheatgrass** is another important food that aids the liver. It also lowers blood pressure, among other numerous health benefits.

Each of these foods will aid certain organs and glands in getting rid of built up toxins in the body. The other health benefits are too numerous to mention, but include prevention of disease, lowering cholesterol levels, boosting immune system and protecting bones and muscles. They should be consumed often, not just for their ability to help the body perform its own cleansing, but for these other health benefits as well.

Q13 ~ What are Signs that a Cleanse is Working?

While some people claim all body cleanses have side effects, others say the side effects are actually proof that the cleanse is doing what it is supposed to and removing toxins from the body. As always, any symptom that becomes acute should be discussed with a physician as soon as possible.

Signs that the body cleanse is working usually last a few days. Skin problems may worsen as the body flushes impurities from the skin and rashes may occur. Other signs to watch for include bad breath, weakness, nausea, headaches, muscle aches, fever, irregular heartbeat, tiredness, dizziness, and dark urine. All of these are signs that toxins are being flushed from the body and that the cleanse is working as it is supposed to.

The more toxins that are built up in the body, the more acute the symptoms of the flushing will be. If a person has a health problem, the symptoms of that health issue may become more acute during a cleanse. Some believe that a healing crisis may happen during a cleanse that mirrors symptoms of past illnesses. Sleeplessness, sinus congestion, fever, and extreme tiredness may all occur while the body is cleansing itself.

To overcome any healing crisis, plenty of water needs to be consumed and the person needs to rest just as if they were recuperating from an illness. Proponents of body cleanses urge people to not give up the cleanse when the symptoms become too uncomfortable as these are signs that the body is actually healing and becoming more healthy. Plenty of liquids and rest should alleviate the discomfort of the healing process.

Peppermint tea may help relieve some of the symptoms, such as upset stomach or headaches. Drinking additional water may also help to flush out the toxins quicker. Anyone who plans to perform a body cleanse needs to choose a time when there will be plenty of time to rest during the cleanse as the person may not feel able to stay in their normal routine.

Total body cleanses can make the body healthier, but flushing the poisons from the body can make anyone feel worse for a few days. If the symptoms do not alleviate quickly, or become too severe, always be sure to contact a physician.

Q14 ~ What is Fasting and How is it a Body Cleanse?

Fasting is a period of time when one abstains from foods and liquids. Fasting can range from abstaining from a certain food or foods, to only drinking liquids, to not ingesting any foods or liquids at all. For thousands of years, people have been fasting to clear their minds and bodies of anything that may be clogging their system. Many religions believe that only through total fasting can a person truly communicate with God. Scientists have offered fasting as a way to heal illnesses and some doctors believe that fasting can cure not only physical pains, but also mental and spiritual problems.

The idea behind fasting is to give the body a break from the everyday need to digest food and eliminate waste. It is believed that fasting gives the body a rest. Much like a vacation gives people a rest from their typical routine and helps recharge their minds and spirits. The withdrawal from food and routine help the body, mind, and spirit reconnect and discover what it really needs.

Fasting is a total body experience. The body, spirit, and mind become more relaxed and less focused on food. Spiritual awareness often heightens and people believe they can let go of painful thoughts from their past when they are fasting. The body cleans out toxins that it cannot remove when food is going through the digestive system. Bad diets can cause a lot of toxins in the body and when fasting, the toxins clean out from the lymph system, colon, blood, kidneys, lungs, sinuses, liver, and skin.

Fasting has become a popular alternative therapy but should be guided by a physician. Anyone who plans to fast longer than 24-48 hours should be under the care of a physician. While some colds and flu may be shortened by a fast, and other medical conditions may be helped, anyone with severe health issues should not consider fasting a safe way to complete a cleanse. People with liver or kidney disease, people with heart problems, diabetics, and pregnant women should avoid fasting. Because medications often require a meal to be eaten to work properly, anyone who takes medication should avoid fasting as well.

Fasting can seem like an easy way to perform a body cleanse. It can be done at home and inexpensively. However, people need to be aware of potential side effects of any type of fasting. Headaches, muscle aches, and nausea may all occur during a fast. Hunger pains can be quite painful. Everyone needs to remember that each body reacts differently to fasting and just because someone else felt amazing and wonderful during their fast does not mean everyone will feel the same way.

The most potentially harmful dangers can occur with long term fasting. These can include a dangerous drop in blood pressure, emotional distress, and persistent cold. If any of these symptoms occur, a fast should be stopped immediately. Other long term effects can include damage to organs and even death. Fasting should not be confused with anorexia, but at times, a person can become hooked on the effects of fasting and become anorexic. Friends and family should carefully monitor anyone who is fasting.

Q15 ~ Are there Pills that can be Used to Cleanse?

There is an almost unlimited number of pills that promise a total body cleanse if they are used. Nearly every health and supplement store has its own name brand of pill and each guarantee that anyone who uses their pill will feel healthier in as little as a few days. It is up to the consumer to choose which one fits their needs and budget. Some of these medicines can be very expensive. Pill regimens can last anywhere from two days to several months depending on the type of pill that is chosen.

Many of the pills that are used for body cleanses can cost anywhere from twenty dollars to well over one hundred. Some pills are for specific body parts, while others are for a total body cleanse. Pills can cause headaches, nausea, and, in some instances, many trips to the bathroom. It is best to be prepared before taking any of them. Carefully read the information that comes with the pills to be sure you are aware of the potential side effects.

The most common side effect of body cleanse pills is stomach cramps. It seems that nearly everyone who consumes these pills will experience stomach cramps of varying degrees. Other side effects that can be felt are weight loss or gain, muscle pain and weakness, sluggishness, and heartburn. Women can develop irregular periods or even no period at all. Both men and women can experience enlarged or tender breasts. Anyone who takes a body cleanse pill can have hives, headaches, nausea, or dizziness. Any of these side effects can become serious. If they become too critical, a visit to a doctor may be needed.

Severe side effects are also possible and if any of these are experienced, a doctor needs to be contacted immediately. These are rare but need to be taken very seriously if any occur. Anyone who becomes uncoordinated or has muscle weakness anywhere in the body needs to see a doctor. An increased risk of bleeding as well as an abnormal heart rhythm is possible. The heart may stop completely or muscle damage may affect the kidneys and cause permanent kidney damage. The central nervous system can be affected and may cause problems with mental alertness.

Anyone who takes daily medication should discuss their body cleanse choice of pills with their doctor before they take any. Many medications will react with others and this can be dangerous.

Even pills that promise they are only herbal medicines should be a concern and warrant a discussion with a physician.

Q16 ~ What are Alternative Ways to Perform Cleanses?

Many people want the results of a body cleanse but are concerned about drastically altering their diet or taking any type of pills. Laxatives are especially concerning to most people as dehydration is a very real possibility. There are ways to remove toxins from the body that do not involve taking any medication, fasting, or changing the diet.

One idea is to try **dry brushing** the skin. Each morning and evening, use a natural bristle brush or a dry loofah to brush the skin. Start at the feet and brush the entire body. This helps to promote lymphatic drainage and encourages the toxins stored under layers of skin to loosen and flush from the body.

Another way to flush toxins from the body is try a **steam bath**. Because it is so relaxing, it helps flush negative thoughts and feelings from the mind and spirit as it encourages toxins to loosen and come out through the skin. Be careful not to get too overheated while enjoying the steam as this may cause dizziness or a lightheaded.

Meditation is another awesome way to cleanse the body. Because the mind, body and spirit are all tied together so closely, relaxing the mind and spirit will also allow toxins to flush from the body. While many believe meditation requires special music or training all that is truly required is a quiet spot where the person feels comfortable and time to relax and turn thoughts to a pleasant place. Some people choose to hold pillows or other soft objects to help keep their focus on the body and to allow negative thoughts to drift away. This is a great way to alleviate stress from everyday life.

Prayer is another option for cleansing the spirit. It does not matter what religion a person is, the ability to sit and quietly talk about any concerns is freeing to many people. It has also been found that giving thanks or listing what they have to be grateful for is a great way for people to lose the negativity in their spirit and help the body remove toxins.

Writing in a journal can also help relax the body and calm the spirit. It has been proven that the stress from everyday life can prevent the body from working as it should to remove toxins. Writing can help quiet the stress and this allows the digestive system of the body to flush out all of the dangerous toxins that seep into the body each day.

Anything a person can do to relax the body, mind or spirit can be used as a body cleanse. Alleviating stress lets the body do its job. Getting enough sleep also helps the body remove toxins. Many experts agree that to get a true cleansing of the body, the mind, spirit and the body all need to be cleansed and rested.

Q17 ~ What is Panchakarma?

Panchakarma is a little known total mind and body cleanse. It was developed in India thousands of years ago and proponents feel it should be completed on a seasonal basis for optimum health of the body and spirit. It can also be completed when a person is feeling ill or just not as healthy as they have been.

This body cleanse assumes that people need to assimilate every aspect of their life that gives them nourishment and to eliminate anything that causes pain or unrest. Stress, unhappiness and anger can allow toxins to gather in the body. This creates an imbalance in the body and toxins will eventually cause illness. Panchakarma is supposed to release any toxins that have been stored in the body and help the body restore its ability to heal.

When the digestive system in the body works as it is supposed to, toxins are quickly removed from the tissues and the body stays healthy. People who believe in the use of Panchakarma feel that negative energy builds up in the body and this prevents the body from cleansing the toxins as easily as it should. Excess fat and high cholesterol are signs of the body not being able to remove some toxins and often, this weight settles around the waist. This can cause blockage of arteries which can lead to heart attacks.

Panchakarma not only helps to heal the body, but also the mind and spirit. Even as the body removes toxins, the mind must be able to remove negative thoughts, such as criticism from a loved one, and also to quiet the spirit and handle negative emotions like anger. The entire body must be in balance for it to be truly healthy and this total body cleansing guarantees it can be done.

The process of Panchakarma is a very detailed one. For several days or weeks, the person must follow a special diet that includes herbs which allows the digestive system to repair itself. While this diet is being used, several types of massages are used to allow the mind and spirit to calm and return to a happy, healthy state. Specific oils are used on the body and applied directly to the forehead to enhance relaxation during the massages.

Each massage is a specially planned movement on the body. Often, two people are giving the massage and they work together to follow the routine and help cleanse the mind and spirit. Again, oils are used to enhance the mental and emotional health of the individual who is receiving Panchakarma. The special massage and oil help release the toxins stored in the body and allow the toxins to return to the digestive system to be flushed from the body.

Steam, with certain herbs infused in it, is also used to encourage the toxins to release from the organs of the body and flow back into the digestive system to be flushed from the body. People who suffer from chronic sinus problems can have herbal oils inserted directly into the nose to aide in flushing allergens from the sinus. This can be a big relief to those who have constant sinus headaches.

The last part of Panchakarma is rejuvenation. Once the toxins have been removed from the body, followers of this body cleanse believe that the energy of the body can be rebuilt. The end result of Panchakarma is a fully functioning digestive system, a relaxed mind and a happy spirit. Followers believe the body is now healed and energy levels are high.

Panchakarma is a very intensive body cleanse and should only be performed by those who understand its power. It needs to be done when the person has plenty of time to rest and relax. A short program lasts about one week and the rejuvenation parts can be finished at home. Some panchakarma programs can last over a month.

This type of total body cleanse can only be performed at a spa or therapeutic center. This is not something that can be completed at home and anyone who would like to try Panchakarma should thoroughly research any clinic that offers this body cleanse. Ask for references and talk to others who have had it done to hear their results and about any side effects they may have experienced.

Q18 ~ What does Traditional Chinese Medicine Believe about Cleanses?

People who follow Traditional Chinese Medicine believe that the body has everything it needs to cleanse itself and that very little should be done to disrupt the natural rhythms of the body. It is believed that every organ in the body has a certain time each day that it cleanses itself. To truly perform the best body cleanse, one must be chosen that works with the body's natural detox routine and not one that disrupts it.

In Chinese medicine, it is very important to choose the right foods to help each organ with its natural cleansing. Chinese herbs can be used as teas to aid the body with cleansing and combining these teas with the right foods will allow the body to cleanse itself even easier and in a natural way that does not disrupt its traditional rhythms.

Traditional Chinese Medicine believes that the health of the body is tied directly to the health of the liver. Part of this tradition is that Qi, the energy that flows through the body, must remain in balance for the body to be healthy. People who follow Chinese medicine support the theory that the liver is the most important organ in the body and that stress, anger, and resentment can all cause the liver and the Qi to become unbalanced. It is believed that each spring, the liver and Qi both need to be cleansed and rebalanced. Many use an ancient process of self-healing to cleanse and rebuild the liver and the Qi to start the New Year healthier and happier.

For the liver, artichokes are one of the best foods to aid in the body's cleansing of that organ. They can be boiled and then eaten either hot or cold. Kidney beans, olive oil, and quinoa are terrific foods to help the body cleanse the kidneys.

Remember, to truly follow a body cleanse from Chinese medicine, the liver is the most important organ of the body and until it is working properly, no other cleanse will be able to produce the benefits of a liver cleansing. Eating foods that help the liver every day will help keep the body healthy.

Q19 ~ Can Massage Really be a Body Cleanse?

Massage can be a great way to detoxify the mind and spirit. Certain types of massage can even help the body rid itself of dangerous toxins. Massage can alleviate symptoms of fibromyalgia and also help with fatigue and headaches. Many people believe that the relaxing effects of massage offers more benefits to the body that any other type of cleanse.

One thing many people like is that massage does not involve consuming any herbs that could be dangerous to people taking medications. They also do not have to make any changes to their diet. Fasting and juice cleanses can have negative effects that massage does not have. For the thousands of people who believe a body cleanse means more than removing toxins from the physical body, a massage is the perfect way to help in the cleanse of the mind and spirit.

A massage therapist will use different techniques to relax the body. Alternating pressure levels and irregular movements stretch and compress muscles to help clear the mind and relax the body. A relaxed body encourages better blood circulation and that allows the liver and kidneys to do their job properly.

There are several types of massages that can help with detoxifying the body. The lymphatic system of the body is the one responsible for removing waste. A specific massage called the lymphatic massage is used to clear dietary toxins from the body. The massage therapist will use certain strokes along the body to encourage the lymphatic system to perform better. It can also remove blockages in the circulatory system. Stress, heavy metals and dead cells can all cause blockages in the system and massage helps to ease these blockages. Experts disagree about whether the massage physically helps the blockages or whether the relaxing effects on the mind actually release blockages.

A massage designed to remove toxins from the body can also help the immune system fight diseases, strengthen muscles, and aid in the connective tissues in the body. A body that is relaxed will function better all around. The repetitive movements of the therapist will also relax the mind and spirit which in turn, let the body relax even more and perform its functions even better. A Swedish massage can also be considered a detoxification process. It helps get oxygen levels to where they are supposed to be and improves the drainage of the elimination organs of the body. A traditional Chinese massage has a different style but the results are the same.

Most health spas offer massages that are designed as a body cleanse. Clients need to request a detoxifying massage when they go for an appointment and many people find the results so amazing they schedule monthly body cleanse massages to go along with a healthier diet and exercise for optimum health benefits and a happier lifestyle.

Q20 ~ What is Purging and is it Harmful to the Body?

Often, when people hear the word "purge" in regards to diet, the first thing they think of is someone who forces themselves to vomit as soon as they eat. This is not exactly what a purge cleanse involves, but it can still be dangerous. While a basic dietary cleanse involves drinking a lot of water and juice, and eating small amounts of food, purging is a quicker way to remove everything from the body. Often, pills or herbs are used to completely flush out the system.

Many purges are diuretics and can dehydrate the body in a very short period of time. Herbal laxatives are also used for purging body cleanses and these can have the same dehydrating effects. Dehydration is extremely dangerous for the human body and purging should only be used in extreme circumstances. At times, purging can be used to remove the lingering effects of an opium-based pain killer from the body, but this should be done under a doctor's care and in a hospital where close monitoring can be done. If you are interested in a purge cleanse it is best to consult a physician for more information.

Q21 ~ Is Exercise Really a Cleanse?

Fitness instructors, yoga instructors, and gyms are often the first to say that exercise is the best way to detoxify the body. Exercise does make people feel better, especially after they get into a routine. Often, people are told that they feel better because they are ridding their bodies of dangerous toxins by exercising and doing certain yoga poses. Experts are not so sure that exercise is actually detoxifying the body.

The kidneys and liver remove toxins from the body, not sweat. Fitness instructors are quick to say that sweat is carrying toxins from the body to encourage people to work out harder and more often. Exercise does help the lungs and, obviously, makes the body healthier. There is little evidence that it actually removes toxins and should be used as a way to enhance a healthy lifestyle. Yoga instructors believe that certain poses squeeze more blood into the kidneys and liver and that is why it is a body cleanse. They believe yoga promotes better blood circulation and that encourages the quicker removal of toxins from the body.

No studies have concluded that exercise truly removes toxins from the body. Instead, a good exercise routine often encourages healthier eating for the participant, which in turn involves eating the very fruits and vegetables that cleanse the body. So while exercise itself may not cleanse the body, the after-effects of the exercise do.

Bonus Q! ~ Is there a Way to Live to Avoid the Need for Total Body Cleanses?

There is a time and place for everything, including total body cleanses. The problem is that people begin relying on cleansing their bodies whenever they feel down or sluggish instead of changing their lifestyle.

To avoid using a body cleanse often, a lifestyle change is in order. Two of the most obvious changes are to stop smoking and to limit alcohol consumption. Neither of these will be popular choices, but for true body health, the changes need to be made. Drinking a lot of water and green tea will help people avoid needing a body cleanse. Water will help the kidneys stay clean and they are one of the major organs in detoxifying the body.

Eat healthier foods. If possible, eat produce that is grown locally as it will be a much healthier choice. If food has to travel great distances, chemicals are sprayed on it to prevent it from spoiling. These chemicals are the very toxins that need to be removed from the body after consumption.

Medications and supplements should be taken in moderation and only as directed by a physician. While these are necessary at times, some of the medications will remain in the body and can cause the need for a body cleanse. Sunshine will also enhance overall health so be sure to get outside as much as possible.

There is no shortcut to perfect health, but each small step that is taken is another step forward in finding a healthy lifestyle. A healthy lifestyle will prevent the need for total body cleanses.

What is the Conclusion to this Book?

Cleansing has been used for thousands of years to help the body fight illnesses, promote healthier living, and even for religious practice. Native Americans believed that only by cleansing their bodies could they calm their spirit and rest their minds enough to communicate with the Gods of their natural world. Ancient Chinese physicians prescribed cleanses to alleviate aches and pains and to prevent new diseases. Even in the modern world, people who believe in alternative medicines use body cleanses to maintain proper health and as a preventative for disease.

In many cases, the benefits can outweigh the dangers of using a body cleanse. It is vital that each person research the type of cleanse they want to use. Many body cleanses just revolve around eating better and adding natural herbs to the diet. The more extreme the cleanse, the more care should be shown by the person who uses it.

With so many options available to try, it may take a few experiments to see what works and whether the cleanse helps you feel any different. A simple body cleanse, such as a juice cleanse, can be performed without a lot of risk and is inexpensive. If a person feels the need for a cleanse, this could be a good way to start.

Thank you for reading. If you enjoyed this book I would greatly appreciate if you posted a review on Amazon. If you send me the link to your review (delightfulpleasuresofficial@gmail.com) I will enter you into a drawing to win a $15 Amazon gift card. This is a continuous drawing I will award every 10 submissions.

Happy Cleansing!

References

Goyanes, Cristina. "Your Guide to Popular Juice Cleanses." 2014. www.health.com

Wallis, Dain. "Natural Ways to Flush Your Toxins without Doing a Cleanse." February 11, 2014. www.huffingtonpost.com

"Why Do a Liver Cleanse and Detox in the Spring?" 2014. www.tcmworld.org

Samuels, Simone. "7 Benefits I Never Expected When I Went on a Raw Foods Diet." MindBodyGreen. July 23, 2014. www.mindbodygreen.com

Imparato, Lauren. "4 Foods to Help Your Body Cleanse." January 1, 2013. www.mindbodygreen.com

www.abesmarket.com

"Panchkarma." 2014. www.chopra.com

"The Master Cleanser Recipe." 2013. www.mastercleanse.com

"Detoxification." 2014. www.wikipedia.org

"Cleansing Symptoms." 2014. www.neera-detox.com

"36 Foods the Help Detox and Cleanse Your
    Entire Body." 2013.
    www.eatlocalgrown.com

Davis, Jeanie. "Detox Diets: Cleansing the Body."
    WebMD. 2002. www.webmd.com

Williams, David Dr. "Probiotic Digestive Health
    and Poor Bacterial Balance. February 6,
    2014.www.drdavidwilliams.com

Zeratsky, Katherine. "Do Detox Diets Offer Any
    Health Benefits?" April 21, 2012.
    www.mayoclinic.org

Grimes, Kelly. "Fasting: Body Cleansing or Body
    Starving?" www.vanderbilt.edu

2014. www.health.howstuffworks.com

"Liver- Anatomy and Function." 2013.
    www.innerbody.com